RHEUMATOID ARTHRITIS "DOCTOR's ADVICE TO PATIENTS"

BLUEPRINT TO PAIN FREE LIFE

By Dr. NIKHIL GUPTA

Table Of Content

COPYRIGHT PAGE

Neither the author nor the publisher can be held responsible for the use of information provided within this book. The decision which a trained professional makes while seeing the patient in person should be the final decision regarding treatment of any patient. Medical science has some limitations, thus individual decisions by a trained professional for each individual patient are different and should be the final decision.

For further information/query – contact drnikhilguptamamc@gmail.com

Website –
http://www.centreforarthritisrheumatologicaldiseases delhi.com

ABOUT THE AUTHOR

I, the author of the book, Dr Nikhil Gupta is a senior consultant rheumatologist practising in Delhi & Haryana, India with a decade of experience. I completed my fellowship in rheumatology and clinical immunology from prestigious Christian Medical College, Vellore, Tamil Nadu and worked department of rheumatology at All India Institute of Medical Sciences, Delhi as senior research fellow. I have many national, international publications and book chapters to my name. I presented my research work in various national and international conferences. I manage patients with rheumatological and autoimmune diseases on daily basis.

Dr. Nikhil Gupta

MD Medicine

Ex fellow rheumatology – CMC Vellore, Tamil Nadu

Ex senior research fellow rheumatology – AIIMS, Delhi

Formerly senior consultant rheumatologist – Max Hospital, Delhi

Director – Centre for Arthritis and Rheumatological Diseases in Delhi

EMail id – drnikhilguptamamc@gmail.com

DEDICATION

I dedicate this book to –

1.   My family who always encouraged me to write a book. I compromised my family time, days, nights & holidays but still my family supported me to write the book for the welfare of the patients.

2.   Secondly, I dedicate this book to my patients who always asked me their queries and many times I found it difficult to answer. Through my patients I realized that treating rheumatoid arthritis is way beyond prescribing medicines. The patients aren't able to identify authentic information about RA. Thus, I got motivated to bridge this gap between doctor and patients with RA.

3.   Life teaches us many things. However, a teacher selflessly guides a student to the path of success and truthfulness. I dedicate this book to my teacher's right from school, medical school, postgraduate, super specialist trainers/mentors (Rheumatologists), colleagues and friends who not only taught me but also guided me to this path.

4.   I also dedicate this book to my patients who constantly motivated me to write this book.

5.   Finally, I dedicate this book to the readers to make full use of its content to improve their quality of life.

INTRODUCTION

This book is written to provide useful information for the patients about rheumatoid arthritis (RA). This book is written by a rheumatologist considering his experience in treating patients. This book contains scientific facts which a patient with RA should know and follow. It answers all the unanswered queries with patients of RA. Educating oneself is the most important thing for a patient of rheumatoid arthritis. Through this book patients shall learn RA symptoms, complications and comorbidities in RA. This book gives a blueprint in managing RA. Patients shall learn to cope up with RA flare and decrease their bad days. This book will help RA patients deal with anxiety and depression, which is commonly seen in RA. Through this book, RA patients would get to know the mistakes which patients make. Patients shall also learn to avoid the side effects of medicines by reading this book. This book gives a blueprint to live a pain free life.

Another interesting thing about this book is why I wrote this book. One of my patients told me one day that not all information is available about the RA, its treatment, lifestyle modifications, medicines & its side effects etc. anywhere. Even if it's available, no one knows the authentic source about it. She requested me to create such information which is available for the patients so that no-one is misled. I was moved by that statement and decided to help patients with the information. I started noting all the queries of my patients and gathered scientific information which is present in this book of mine. It took a huge effort to create such an information source.

This book gives a holistic approach for the management of RA and contains the blueprint to live a pain free life.

To the best of my knowledge, this book on RA is the only book written by a rheumatologist (a specialist who treats RA) for the patients in such a great detail.

I wish the patients with RA- a healthy, prosperous and pain free life.

CHAPTER 1

RHEUMATOID ARTHRITIS OVERVIEW

WHAT IS RHEUMATOID ARTHRITIS?
Rheumatoid arthritis (RA) is an autoimmune disease in which the patient's immune system mistakenly attacks its own body thinking as foreign. It is a chronic inflammatory disease that can affect joints and other organs of the body like heart, brain, kidneys, lungs, eyes, etc. RA is the most common inflammatory joint disease, seen in 1-2% of the population around the world. The inflammation associated with rheumatoid arthritis can affect major organs of the body like skin, eyes, lungs, heart, kidneys, nerves and blood vessels. With the advent of new medicines, a patient with rheumatoid arthritis stands a good chance to live a normal to near normal life.

RISK FACTORS OF RHEUMATOID ARTHRITIS
Factors which increase risk of developing RA are -

1.   Age - RA can begin at any age, though commonly it occurs in middle age.
2.   Sex - RA typically affects females, two-to-three times higher than men.
3.   Genes - People whose body contain specific genes such as HLA (human leukocyte antigen) are more likely to develop RA.
4.   Family History – Those with a family history of RA are at increased risk of developing the same. The risk is not 100 %, however a small increase as compared to the general population.

5.   Smoking – Smoking is an established risk factor for RA. Smoking makes the disease worse and increases risk of lung development in RA.

6.   Obesity - Being obese increases the risk of developing RA

7.   Environment – Chemical exposure or certain viral infections increase the risk of developing RA

8.   Diet -   Drinking sugary soda on a regular basis increases the risk of developing rheumatoid arthritis

Taking care of dental hygiene helps control inflammation associated with rheumatoid arthritis. Thus, good dental health can help control RA.

SYMPTOMS OF RHEUMATOID ARTHRITIS –

Rheumatoid arthritis can have varied manifestations. Its manifestations define the symptoms which a patient can develop. Common symptoms of RA include:

•   Pain, stiffness or swelling in one or more joint
•   Weight loss
•   Fever
•   Fatigue, weakness or tiredness

Symptoms may vary depending on the organ involved. For example – a patient may have red eyes, dryness in the eyes (gritty feeling), dry mouth, dry skin, dry cough, rashes over skin etc.

HOW IS RHEUMATOID ARTHRITIS DIAGNOSED?

RA is a clinical diagnosis, diagnosed by typical symptoms and signs after examining a patient with supportive evidence from lab tests. Tests like ESR and CRP may be raised in patients with RA, especially at the time of disease activity. Rheumatoid factor and/or anti CCP levels are generally raised in patients with RA, but may be in normal range in 30-40 percent patients. So, a negative Rheumatoid factor or anti CCP levels does not rule out its diagnosis.

RHEUMATOID ARTHRITIS – WHICH ALL ORGANS CAN IT INVOLVE?
Rheumatoid arthritis can have extra articular (involvement other than joints) manifestations in about 40% of patients. These manifestations can occur either in the beginning or anytime during the course of their disease.
Cimmino MA, Salvarani C, Macchioni P. Extra-articular manifestations in 587 Italian patients with rheumatoid arthritis. Rheumatol Int. 2000;19(6):213–217.
These manifestations are more common in patients with active and severe RA. Thus, early aggressive approach shall seem to be appropriate in view of the adverse effect of extra articular manifestations on RA outcomes. Rheumatoid arthritis is associated with a high risk of morbidity and premature death secondary to the earlier development of cardiovascular, lung diseases and malignancy.
Crostein BN. Interleukin-6 – a key mediator of systemic and local symptoms in rheumatoid arthritis. Bull NYU Hosp J Dis. 2007;65(Suppl 1):S11–S15.

Extra articular involvement in RA includes –
1.   Skin

2.   Eyes
3.   Mouth (oral)
4.   Lungs
5.   Cardiac (heart)
6.   Kidneys
7.   Neurological
8.   Hematological (blood)

SKIN INVOLVEMENT

Rheumatoid nodules (lumps over bone or skin) are the most frequent skin manifestations in RA. They are seen in around 20% of patients with RA. Rheumatoid vasculitis (swelling of blood vessels) can be seen on the skin. It may manifest in the form of haemorrhages (red spots on skin), ulcers over the leg and gangrene of fingers. The patient may have dry skin as the manifestation due to the secondary sjogren syndrome.

EYE INVOLVEMENT

The most frequent eye manifestation is dry eyes seen in around 10-15% patients with RA. Sometimes, it may be the first manifestation of RA. Other manifestations of eyes in RA include – red eyes, which can be painless or painful. Rarely, ulcers can develop in the eyes, which can lead to corneal melt.

ORAL MANIFESTATIONS

Dry mouth can be a manifestation of patients with RA. Decreased production of saliva can lead to dental caries. Patients with RA who develop dental caries have aggressive disease, difficult to control with medicines. A proper treatment of dental caries can solve this problem.

LUNG MANIFESTATION

Lung involvement may occur in the form of interstitial lung disease which may manifest as a dry cough. Patients with RA have increased risk of being asthmatics which may manifest as wheezing, breathing difficulty with or without cough. There may be nodules in the lungs. Patients with RA are at high risk of acquiring lung infections as pneumonia, tuberculosis, etc.

CARDIAC DISEASE

The risk for heart attack in female patients with RA is twice that of a normal healthy female. In long-standing disease of at least 10 years, the risk of heart attack is 3 times higher as compared to the general population. Patients with RA more often develop heart failure than those with normal healthy populations. Heart involvement in RA increases the risk of premature death.

KIDNEY INVOLVEMENT

Kidney involvement in RA is uncommon. Rarely, inflammation in the kidneys can lead to protein leakage.

NEUROLOGICAL MANIFESTATIONS

Nerve involvement is common in RA patients. The patient may feel numbness, burning, paresthesias, weakness of hands or feet. When a nerve of hand (median nerve) is affected, it is called carpal tunnel syndrome. It may manifest as involvement of a joint between the skull and spinal cord which, if severe, can lead to paralysis.

HEMATOLOGICAL (BLOOD) INVOLVEMENT

RA may lead to low haemoglobin, increase in platelets and low leukocyte count. RA increases the risk of blood cancers as lymphoma or leukemia.

PSYCHIATRIC MANIFESTATIONS

RA is associated with psychosomatic manifestations as anxiety and depression. Depression and anxiety in RA patients have poor treatment outcomes.

CONCLUSION

Although RA is considered a "joint disease" it can involve major organs of the body known as extra articular manifestations. The prevalence of these manifestations is about 40% of RA patients. Extra articular involvement is more common in men, smokers, more severe joint disease, irregular treatment and worse function. The longer the duration of the disease will be, the larger the number of extra-articular manifestations and are associated with worse outcomes.

CHAPTER 2

COMPLICATIONS AND COMORBIDITIES IN RHEUMATOID ARTHRITIS

Untreated, long standing or improperly controlled rheumatoid arthritis patients are bound to develop complications and comorbidities. The same may develop in controlled disease as well as in early disease but the percentage is much less in such cases.

COMPLICATIONS IN RHEUMATOID ARTHRITIS

Most of the patients think that rheumatoid arthritis is a disease of the joints. As described earlier, it can affect many organ systems in the body. Just like swelling/inflammation in the joints, RA can cause inflammation in major organs of the body thus leading to damage and RA related complications. RA related complications are -

1.   Joint Damage –

Rheumatoid arthritis if not treated early or not well controlled can lead to joint damage, which may require surgery. Inflammation or joint swelling can damage the joint cartilage, tendons and nearby bone. This may lead to joint deformities and disabilities.

2.   Osteoporosis-

Osteoporosis means weak bones thus leading to increase in risk of fracture. Osteoporosis in RA is majorly due to Rheumatoid arthritis itself, along with some contribution from medications used in its treatment. The lifetime risk of developing fracture is as high as 40% in patients who develop osteoporosis in RA.

3.   Infections –

Patients with RA are at increased risk of mild to life threatening infections. The risk of infection is highest when the disease is active. Risk of infection is contributed more by the disease activity then by medicines used to treat the disease barring a few infections. Vaccines are recommended to prevent infections in RA.

4.   Abnormal body composition -

Patients of RA have higher fat to lean mass ratio, even in people who have a normal body mass index (BMI). Patients with RA lose muscle mass but regain fat which predisposes the patient to cardiovascular diseases.

5.   Heart problems –
Rheumatoid arthritis increases the risk of hardening and blockage of arteries. Patients with RA have high risk of developing cardiovascular disease. There is increased risk of getting heart attack, stroke and heart failure. Smoking, obesity, comorbidity like diabetes, deranged body cholesterol and increased blood pressure, unhealthy diet and inadequate exercise are risk factors in addition to uncontrolled rheumatoid arthritis which further increase the risk of cardiovascular disease.

6.   Lung disease –
People with rheumatoid arthritis have an increased risk of inflammation and shrinkage of the lung. This can lead to dry cough and progressive shortness of breath. People with RA are at increased risk of developing lung infections as pneumonia, tuberculosis, etc.

7.   Lymphoma -
Rheumatoid arthritis increases the risk of blood cancer as lymphoma. Some studies point out that patients with RA have increased risk of developing lung, liver and esophageal cancer.

8.   Memory Loss, Anxiety & depression –
Memory loss, anxiety and depression are common in patients with rheumatoid arthritis seen in almost two third of patients. Patients may feel uneasiness, lack of sleep, palpitations, ghabrahat, negative feelings or thought and forgetfulness. These manifestations may lead to skipping medicines and increase in pain.

IS RHEUMATOID ARTHRITIS CURABLE?

RA is a long term disease requiring long term treatment, but this should not frighten the patient. Just like hypertension, thyroid diseases, diabetes, heart diseases etc RA too require lifelong treatment. Just like hypertension and diabetes, regular treatment if started early should control the disease and prevent deformities and disabilities. Long term studies reveal that 10-14% of patients of early RA (disease duration less than 2 years) go into long term remission (absence of any sign & symptoms) without medicines.

ARE RA PATIENTS AT RISK OF PREMATURE DEATH?

RA is mostly considered a disease of only joints by most people. They think that this disease won't affect their life span as it only affects their joints. However, this is not true. Inflammation occurs in each and every part of the body just like swelling in the joints.

• Lifespan of an RA patient is 10-15 years shorter than average normal
• However, RA patients whose disease have been under control - may have normal life expectancy
• Factors shown to reduce life span – cardiovascular disease, respiratory involvement as ILD, Obstructive airway disease, infections as pneumonia, musculoskeletal condition as deformities
Complications that determines the life span of patients with RA –
• how far RA has progressed
• sex, with females (chance of severe RA is more)

- early diagnosis and treatment associated with minimal complications and favorable outcomes
- individual risk factors, as a family history of heart disease, diabetes
- Smoking and drinking alcohol have been associated with decreased life span
- Medications – disease-modifying antirheumatic drugs (methotrexate, sulfasalazine, hydroxychloroquine, leflunomide) and biologics reduce the risk of complications
- Early diagnosis and treatment - controls inflammation - reduces the risk of death

COMORBIDITIES IN RHEUMATOID ARTHRITIS

Comorbidities in RA patients are increased as compared to the general population. Comorbidities increase in RA patients as RA causes inflammation in all organs of the body from head to toe. On an average, RA patients have two or more co morbid conditions.

Michaud K, Wolfe F. Comorbidities in rheumatoid arthritis. Best Pract Res Clin Rheumatol. 2007;21(5):885-906. doi:10.1016/j.berh.2007.06.002

These co morbid conditions increase the risk of premature death in RA patients.

Dougados M, Soubrier M, Perrodeau E et al. Impact of a nurse-led programme on comorbidity management and impact of a patient self-assessment of disease activity on the management of rheumatoid arthritis: results of a prospective, multicentre, randomised, controlled trial (COMEDRA). Ann. Rheum. Dis. 74(9), 1725–1733 (2015).

Comorbidities associated with RA are cardiovascular disease (heart attack, paralysis or stroke), cancers (breast, blood, lung, skin and rectal); complications related to infections (influenza, pneumonia), diabetes, increased blood pressure and deranged blood cholesterol. Prevalence of comorbidities in patients with RA varies between 40 and 66%.

Daien. Assessment of comorbidities in rheumatoid arthritis. Revue. De. Medicine. Interne. 40, 40-43 (2019).

HOW TO REDUCE COMORBIDITIES IN RA

Dedicated and motivated patients always find it easy to manage RA and comorbidities.

Ways to reduce the comorbidities in RA are -

1. Control RA – Early control of RA along with regular check up with a rheumatologist reduces the risk of developing comorbidities.

2. Regular blood test – Routine blood test ordered by your doctor aims to detect any development of comorbidities. Detecting early and starting medicines helps control the disease, thus preventing complications.

3. Weight loss – Weight loss in an obese or over weight patient reduces the risk of development of comorbidity.

4. Diet control – Reducing sweets, sugar, soda, soft drinks, fried food and fast food helps reduce the risk of developing comorbidities in RA patients. If a patient with RA already has developed comorbidities, diet control can help reduce or control the comorbidities.

5.   Regular exercise – Regular exercise not only controls RA symptoms, but also helps reduce the risk or controls comorbidities.

CHAPTER 3
SEXUAL HEALTH IN RHEUMATOID ARTHRITIS

Sexuality and its expression are important for healthy and ill individuals and play an important part in an individual's self-identity.

Sexual functioning is a neglected area of quality of life in patients with RA that is neither discussed by patients or doctors. RA may affect all aspects of life, including sexual health. RA patients could experience diminished sexual drive due to body and joint pain. The factors which affect sexual functioning in RA are joint pain or stiffness, tiredness, functional impairment like deformities, depression, anxiety, negative body image due to deformities, reduced desire for sex, hormonal imbalance and involvement of organs like heart, lungs. About 31-76% of arthritis patients experience sexual problems.

1.   Gordon D, Beastall GH, Thomson JA, Sturrock RD. Androgenic status and sexual function in males with rheumatoid arthritis and ankylosing spondylitis. Q J Med 1986; 60: 671-679 [PMID: 3094090]
2.   Kraaimaat FW, Bakker AH, Janssen E, Bijlsma JW. Intrusiveness of rheumatoid arthritis on sexuality in male and female patients living with a spouse. Arthritis Care Res 1996; 9: 120-125 [PMID: 8970270]

Sexual function disturbances can occur before, during and after sexual activities. Thus RA can affect sexual health in a negative way. Manifestations of sexual disability include - difficulty in assuming certain positions due to arthritis of hip or knee joint limiting movements, painful intercourse due to vaginal dryness and fatigue during intercourse.

Below is a tablet that shows sexual dysfunction in RA patients, what factors lead to such dysfunction and how patients can improve the sexual functions. Patients should discuss their sexual health with their doctor and can find solutions for the same.

Sexual dysfunction	Factors	Recommendations for patients
1. Sexual disability	Limited mobility, pain, fatigue, morning stiffness	Change position, analgesic intake, heat and muscle relaxation before activity
2. Painful intercourse	Vaginal dryness	Vaginal lubrication,

		estrogen cream
3. Decreased desire	Anxiety, depression	Counselling, antidepressant medicines after consulting a doctor
4. Impotence	Hormonal imbalance	Sidenafil, sex therapy in consultation with a doctor

Some general recommendations to improve sexual functioning in RA include - discussion of the problems with the partner specially the partner's fear of causing pain during sexual intercourse. Patients should explore different positions, use analgesic medicines (if no contraindications), heat therapy and muscle relaxants medicines before sexual activity. These recommendations help improve sexual health in patients with rheumatoid arthritis.

CHAPTER 4

RHEUMATOID ARTHRITIS DURING PREGNANCY AND LACTATION

Rheumatoid arthritis is a disease which can affect young females of reproductive age group. Due to this age group, pregnancy and lactation are two most important phases where this disease can make an impact in a female's life. Controlling rheumatoid arthritis is the most important factor before a patient plans pregnancy. During pregnancy, RA gets subdued in most of the patients. However, in some it may get flared up. RA gets flared up post delivery in most of the patients.

Medicines used to treat RA need to be changed during pregnancy and lactation. All medicines are not safe during these special circumstances. There are many medicines which need to be stopped well in advance before planning pregnancy. A patient must consult his/her doctor before planning pregnancy, during pregnancy and lactation on a regular basis. Patients may require some supplements during pregnancy and lactation, which shall be best answered by the treating doctor.

CHAPTER 5

COURSE OF RHEUMATOID ARTHRITIS

Rheumatoid arthritis is a complex disease. Its natural course is variable in patients. For some it may be a mild disease hardly requiring medicines. However, for some it may be a nightmare as the disease may be so severe which hardly responds to any medicines. Course of RA varies from patient to patient and is described below -

•   According to studies, RA may get cured in 10-14% of patients, especially in those where it is detected and treated early.
•   15-20 percent of patients have intermittent disease with periods of exacerbation and a relatively good prognosis..
•   Some have periods of worsening symptoms that alternate with periods of remission
•   Most patients experience, progressive disease (may progress slowly or quickly) and damage the bones, cartilage, and other structures of the joints
•   Joint damage typically worsens over time and is irreversible and impact's person's routine activities, and lead to significant disability
•   RA can involve major organs of the body like heart, brain, kidney & lungs
•   Deformities don't develop in regularly, however treated patients, however untreated or irregularly treated patient's will develop deformities and require surgeries

- Regularly treated patients live normal to near normal quality of life, however, it is poor in irregular or untreated patients
- Life expectancy is near normal in regularly treated patients however in untreated or irregular treated it is 15 years short

CHAPTER 6

ECONOMIC BURDEN DUE TO RHEUMATOID ARTHRITIS

Rheumatoid arthritis, not only affects a person physically, but also drains him/her financially. It increases the economic burden to the diseased person, but also to the family and even society. RA is associated with increased comorbidities like diabetes, increased blood pressure, heart attacks, stroke and deranged cholesterol. These comorbidities increase the economic burden among patients with RA. Studies concluded RA causes significant economic burden not only for patients but as well the society. In developed nations such as the USA, Canada and the UK, where most of the direct cost is covered under insurance, work-related disabilities and sick leaves cost the economy some billions of dollars. A study reported that over a period of 10 years, arthritis related work loss has been associated with a 37% drop in income. By comparison, people without arthritis had a 90% rise in income over the same period of time.

The economic burden of RA patients is associated with the direct and indirect costs of the disease. Direct costs associated with rheumatoid arthritis is defined by the process used in direct patient care which includes –

1. Professional fee
2. Medication

3.   Diagnostic
4.   Hospitalization
5.   Surgeries
6.   Transportation

These costs are country specific, generally being high in developed countries and low to moderate in developing nations.

Indirect costs take into account the reduced earning capacity and decreased life expectancy. Indirect cost is difficult to estimate. Considering the age of onset of RA and disabilities associated with it, indirect cost outweighs the direct cost of RA.

Thus, RA significantly increases the economic burden among patients with RA.

WAYS TO DECREASE THE COST OF TREATMENT

Ways to reduce the cost are
1.   Early treatment
2.   Regular follow up
3.   Regular exercise
4.   Weight reduction
5.   Controlling co-morbidities

Starting treatment early will prevent deformities and disabilities and hence prevent surgeries. Early treatment will control disease early and won't require costly medicines in most patients. Thus, a patient can easily work throughout their life without affecting their professional life. This shall prevent both direct and indirect expenses.

Regular follow up will help in early detection of any complication be it due to disease or medicines. Thus an early intervention by the doctor will reverse those complications thus preventing hospitalisation and saving cost.

CHAPTER 7

RHEUMATOID ARTHRITIS FLARE & ITS MANAGEMENT

DEFINITION

•	Flares are intermittent bouts of increased rheumatoid arthritis disease activity causing fatigue, flu like symptoms, pain, swelling and stiffness in joints
•	Other symptoms associated with it – sleep disturbance, generalized body pain, difficulty in doing day to day work

CAUSES OF RA FLARE

Some known causes are –

1.	STRESS – Stress is a known trigger for many diseases and RA is no exception.
2.	INFECTIONS – as mild as the common cold can increase RA disease activity.
3.	FOODS – Exact culprit is difficult to pinpoint as problematic food is different for different patients. Patients can list down food which doesn't suit them and should avoid those foods.
4.	OVER EXERTION – Over exertion is associated with an increase in RA disease activity.
5.	POST DELIVERY - Pregnancy is associated with an altered immune system. Post delivery, the immune system tends to return to normal but sometimes it becomes rogue leading to a flare of arthritis.

6.   HORMONAL DISTURBANCE – Rheumatoid arthritis is more common in females. Female hormonal factors are implicated as a causative factor. Hormonal imbalance is also implicated in a flare of RA.

7.   INJURIES – Any injury can trigger a flare of RA.

8.   SMOKING – Smoking is implicated both as a causative agent as well as a cause of flare.

9.   POLLUTION – Air and water pollutants are being postulated as a risk factor for flare of RA.

Many causes are still unknown and research is being carried out to know other factors which lead to flare of RA.

LAB TESTS MAY SUGGEST DISEASE FLARE OR DISEASE ACTIVITY IN RA

Rheumatoid activity disease activity is gauged by a combination of symptoms and inflammatory markers like ESR and CRP. However, ESR and CRP are not sensitive or specific markers of disease activity in RA. These markers may be raised due to multiple other factors. Many times these markers may be normal despite the high disease activity. Thus, it has to be a combination of symptoms and signs along with correct interpretation of inflammatory markers by a treating doctor that determines the disease activity in RA.

•   A flare of RA may lead to severe pain, disturbance, sleepless nights, absent from work and monetary loss.

•   It shall slowly but surely lead to joint damage.

•   So it is essential to identify the symptoms (as mentioned above) early.

MEASURES TO CONTROL FLARE

• Patients with RA should bath with lukewarm water which shall decrease pain and stiffness.
• Patients with RA flare should reduce/manage stress, which can be done through meditation, yoga, engaging in a relaxing hobby, talking to a friend or relative.
• Inadequate sleep increases RA symptoms and hence precipitates flare. Thus, patients with RA should take adequate sleep which, decreases the risk of RA flare. Adequate sleep during a flare also helps decrease RA symptoms.
• There are certain foods which can flare RA. However, these foods are difficult to identify. Patients should avoid canned juices and beverages, sugary food and processed carbohydrates. These foods induce inflammation in the body and hence can precipitate a flare.
• Smoking is a risk factor for RA. It is also a risk factor for the flare of RA. Patients with RA who smoke are at risk of lung involvement, severe RA joint symptoms, risk of heart attacks and stroke. Similarly, patients who smoke are at increased risk of recurrent flare.

Patients should visit their doctor as soon as possible so that he adds some medicines to control flare. Controlling flare early will help reduce pain and swelling early and prevent absent from work.

In spite of all these measures, one can still have a flare, but the number of flares shall decrease and flares shall be mild or less severe.

.

CHAPTER 8

EMOTIONAL AND PSYCHOLOGICAL ASPECTS IN RHEUMATOID ARTHRITIS AND ITS MANAGEMENT

Rheumatoid arthritis is a common disease which affects many people in the world. RA can affect any organ of the body including heart, kidneys, lung, liver, nerves, eye etc. If not treated, these diseases can be fatal. Rheumatologists are specialists who are trained to treat them best.

Mental health comprises emotional and psychological well being. Psychological issues including depression, mood changes and anxiety are common in patients with arthritis and autoimmune diseases. A study (Jacob et al. Depression Risk in Patients with Rheumatoid Arthritis in the United Kingdom. Rheumatol Ther 2017;4, 195–200) conducted in Britain found that within 5 years of RA diagnosis, about 30-35 percent of patients develop depression. Another emotional state commonly seen in patients of RA is anxiety, which is seen in 21% to 70%.

According to the research at Mayo Clinic, untreated depression and psychological issues can make it harder to treat Rheumatoid arthritis. Such patients tend to skip medicines due to depression. It may also affect personal relationships and work performance. These patients are more susceptible to repeated recurrence of intense pain. Thus it is as important to treat arthritis as is your mental health.

HOW TO ATTAIN EMOTIONAL AND PSYCHOLOGICAL WELLBEING IN PATIENTS SUFFERING FROM RHEUMATOID ARTHRITIS?

There are many other aspects which need to be taken care of. A holistic approach is required for treatment of such disease. These measures decrease the dependence on medicines and act as adjunct in the management of RA. I would be explaining about all such issues under various headings as below -

a)   HOW TO IDENTIFY EMOTIONAL WELL BEING IN RHEUMATOID ARTHRITIS
b)   MANAGING PSYCHOLOGICAL ASPECTS AND NEGATIVE THINKING IN RHEUMATOID ARTHRITIS
c)   STRESS MANAGEMENT IN RHEUMATOID ARTHRITIS
d)   IMPORTANCE OF BALANCED LIFE IN MANAGING PSYCHOLOGICAL AND EMOTIONAL ASPECTS IN PATIENTS OF RHEUMATOID ARTHRITIS
e)   ROLE OF REFRESHING SLEEP, DIET AND EXERCISE IN MANAGING PSYCHOLOGICAL AND EMOTIONAL ASPECTS IN RHEUMATOID ARTHRITIS

1. IDENTIFICATION OF EMOTIONAL AND PSYCHOLOGICAL WELL BEING -

When you feel down, worry or think excessively, these feelings can many a time limit your ability to look after yourself. It may limit your ability to manage your arthritis. It may affect your emotional health. Pain, mental health and disability are strongly linked. Recognizing your symptoms is the first and most important step.

The questions below shall help you identify emotional and psychological wellness -

- Are you happy or feel sad?
- Are you enjoying life or not?
- Do you feel tired even at rest?
- Do you have refreshing sleep?

If your response is negative then you are emotionally and psychologically disturbed.

2. MANAGING PSYCHOLOGICAL ASPECTS AND NEGATIVE THINKING IN PATIENTS OF RHEUMATOID ARTHRITIS

Negative thinking can lead to depression, anxiety, fear or hopelessness.

Negative thinking shall be controlled by following techniques –

a) VISUALIZING SOLUTION –

Visualize yourself that you have come out of the task you were going to perform. This will imbibe positive energy in you. You would certainly perform your task with calm and ease.

b) POSITIVE SELF TALK –

To defeat the negative thinking, you need to talk to yourself positively. Think opposite of the negative though you get.

Example - If you get negative thoughts that you are not going to go shopping – just keep telling yourself that I will be able to go shopping.

c)   PSYCHOLOGIST   OR   PSYCHIATRIST APPOINTMENT –

However, if your symptoms are severe or not getting controlled with the above measures tell your treating doctor or ask for a referral to a psychiatrist or psychologist. In addition to the above measures, many patients would require medications for management of their psychological symptoms.

3.   STRESS MANAGEMENT IN RHEUMATOID ARTHRITIS

Stress is a risk factor for many diseases like hypertension, diabetes, heart diseases etc. Stress also precipitates arthritis and autoimmune diseases. It may also lead to fibromyalgia or chronic pain syndrome.

One must take all the measures to reduce stress so as to prevent above mentioned diseases. I will stress upon some measures to reduce stress.

Stress buster techniques –

a)   MEDITATION
Meditation is a technique that if practiced for at least
10 minutes per day, can help control stress and
decrease anxiety. Patients of fibromyalgia performing
meditation daily shall benefit. Reducing stress levels
will not only lower the risk of cardiovascular diseases
but also prevent flare of arthritis and development of
chronic pain syndrome.

b)   JACOBSON'S RELAXATION TECHNIQUE
Jacobson's relaxation technique focuses on
tightening and relaxing specific muscle groups in
sequence. This technique involving the muscles
could relax the mind as well. The technique involves
tightening one muscle group while keeping the rest of
the body relaxed, and then releasing the tension on
that muscle. It helps in dealing with anxiety and is
one of the known treatment options for chronic pain
syndrome or fibromyalgia.

c)   RELAXATION ACTIVITIES
Sitting in a park, watching T.V., movies etc will help
decrease stress and help in controlling stress.

d)   TIME MANAGEMENT
If one manages time properly, stress would decrease
automatically.
Some ways to manage time –
            Schedule everything
            Give some time to your bed/ rest
            Prioritize your work

e)   SOCIAL SUPPORT

Family and friends are great support to an individual. Meeting them makes your mind and body relax. Attending functions and parties can make people shed off stress.

4.   BALANCED LIFE

People focus on work and more work thus losing a balance in life. Restoring work life balance helps reduce stress, anxiety and depression. People should prioritize life and should focus on main goals in life. To live a balanced life, one should focus on –

a)   Career development and growth
b)   Personal development and learning
c)   Social growth and development
d)   Physical growth and development

A person who is living a balanced life shall lead a stressful life.

Mild to moderate emotional and psychological issues are easily managed by the above measures. However, patients may require psychiatrist referral or medications in early disease. Kindly tell your symptoms to your treating doctor who will guide whether or not medications are needed for emotional and psychological support.

5.   ROLE OF REFRESHING SLEEP, DIET AND EXERCISE IN MANAGING EMOTIONAL AND PSYCHOLOGICAL ASPECTS IN RHEUMATOID ARTHRITIS

Sleep, diet and exercise play an important role in managing arthritis as well as psychological and emotional aspects in patients of rheumatoid arthritis.

a)   REFRESHING SLEEP

Studies show that as many as 80% of people with rheumatoid arthritis have sleeping issues. Most of the patients do not sleep properly or don't have refreshing sleep or feel tired when they wake up. Patients often attribute sleep problems to pain however sleep, pain and inflammation go hand in hand and it's a multi directional relationship between them. Those patients who don't get proper sleep often land up in depression or anxiety disorders. Sleep disturbance increases the arthritis and autoimmune disease by increasing inflammation in the body.

Ways to normalize your sleep -

Relaxation exercise like meditation, deep breathing, Jacobson's relaxation technique

Avoiding day time sleep

Sleep hygiene - having a quiet sleep environment, avoid caffeine, other stimulants, nicotine, alcohol, excessive fluids, or stimulating activities before bedtime

Cognitive behavior therapy, biofeedback therapy, paradoxical intention therapy as taught by a psychologist or psychiatrist

Medications prescribed by psychiatrist or physician

Thus it is very important to talk to your treating doctor about sleep so that he manages your rheumatoid arthritis better.

b) DIET

Several studies have shown strong correlations between a healthy diet and mental well-being. Diet rich in fresh fruits and vegetables is linked with increased happiness and better mental health and well-being. There are many studies which prove that patients who eat Mediterranean diet rich in omega fatty acid, fruits and vegetables are less prone to anxiety and depression.

There are studies which show that nutritional deficiencies like vitamins and minerals lead to dementia and depression. Deficiencies of vitamin B12, thiamine, niacin, vitamin D and folic acid lead to poor brain and nerve development and shall lead to depression, anxiety and emotional lability. Thus, taking care of all these aspects of diet and nutrition can help improve emotional imbalance; reduce stress, anxiety and depression.

c) EXERCISE

Physical activity and exercise can partially prevent and improve symptoms of depression, anxiety, low mood and emotional imbalance. Depression and anxiety leads to increases in inflammatory response. Physical activity and exercise training help in increasing anti-inflammatory response and thus control depression and anxiety.

Exercise and physical activity can confer protection from depression at all ages. In patients with anxiety and depression, exercise and physical activity is useful in controlling its symptoms.

One should also consult his treating doctor for the above advice before starting these manures.

CONCLUSION

To conclude – medications need to be complemented and supplemented by diet, exercise, balanced lifestyle, stress management, controlling negative thoughts and relaxation exercise. All these things together shall control psychological and emotional aspects in arthritis and autoimmune disease.

CHAPTER 9

ROLE OF EXERCISE, JOINT PROTECTION MANEUVERS & ACTIVITIES OF DAILY LIVING IN PATIENTS WITH RHEUMATOID ARTHRITIS

Rheumatoid arthritis is a chronic disease requiring lifelong treatment. Treatment goals include pain relief and slow down the activity of RA to prevent deformity, disability and increase functional capacity of the patient.

ROLE OF EXERCISE IN PATIENTS WITH RHEUMATOID ARTHRITIS

Most RA patients suffer from an accelerated loss of muscle mass which contributes to disability and worsens the quality of life of patients. In addition, RA is associated with increased morbidity and death from cardiovascular disease. It has been found that RA patients do less exercise than their healthy people. The physical inactivity of RA patients is a vicious circle in the way of health and disease progression.

Exercise helps patients cope with chronic pain and disability by increasing flexibility, endurance, range of motion (ROM), muscle & bone strength, bone integrity, and prevents cardiovascular disease, coordination and balance. Research has shown that exercise helps to relieve symptoms of rheumatoid arthritis. However, one should talk to his/her doctor before starting an exercise program. Patients can incorporate a mix of flexibility, range of motion, aerobic and strengthening exercises.

BENEFITS OF EXERCISE IN RA INCLUDES -
- Protect the joint from further damages
- Provide pain relief
- Prevent deformity disability
- Increase functional capacity
- Improve flexibility and strength
- Increase range of motion
- Improve general fitness
- Prevent/Improves heart diseases, diabetes and other problems
- Improves emotional and mental well being

Which exercises a patient of RA should do?
- Gentle physical exercise
- Aerobic exercise like swimming, walking, cycling (only if his/her body is fit enough)
- Strengthening exercise as light weight training
- Generalized stretching and range of motion exercises

WHICH EXERCISES ARE FEASIBLE FOR ACUTE PHASE (DURING JOINT PAIN & SWELLING) IN RA

- Perform exercise at least once a day
- Gentle assisted movement through normal range (joint Mobilisation) should be done at all the joints
- Isometric " static muscle contraction" helps to maintain muscle tone without increasing inflammation

WHICH EXERCISES SHOULD BE DONE DURING CHRONIC PHASE (NO/MILD JOINT PAIN OR SWELLING) IN RA

1. Light resistance exercises should be performed
2. Postural / core stability exercises should be performed
3. If your body permits, swimming, walking, cycling should be done to maintain cardiovascular fitness
4. Gentle stretches for areas that become tight, such as knees & calves should be performed

ROLE OF YOGA IN RHEUMATOID ARTHRITIS

Yoga is a practice that includes poses, breathing techniques and meditation. It started in ancient India and is thought as a way to boost physical and mental health. Yoga has shown to help people with arthritis improve many physical symptoms like pain and stiffness, and psychological issues like stress and anxiety. People with various types of arthritis who practice yoga regularly can reduce joint pain, improve joint flexibility and function, and lower stress and tension to promote better sleep.

JOINT PROTECTION IN PATIENTS OF RHEUMATOID ARTHRITIS

In 60% of RA patient's functional ability decreases within the first five years from diagnosis and within two years 50% patients experience difficulties in household tasks.

Joint protection is a self-management technique that helps maintain functional ability of joints by changing working methods of affected joints. This can be done with the help of certain devices such as splints, modified utensils or modifying the movements. Thus, changing the working methods can reduce pain and stress that is applied to the joints during daily activities. These joint protection techniques reduce the wear & tear in the joints and hence prevent joint damage. By modifying work methods and environments, use of assistive devices (assistive technologies) and inclusion of breaks in the routine, pain can be reduced both at rest and motion. Strengthening the peri articular muscles and maintaining joint range of motion by exercise, also contribute in a big way to the maintenance or improvement of the patient's functional capacity.

Joint protection techniques include –
1.   PLANNING
Proper planning before doing a work can minimize the effort and give maximum output.
a.   Do the maximum work at that time of the day when you have minimum or no pain.
b.   Try to do some work online example- paying bills.
c.   Start with more difficult tasks.
d.   Break the workload and take rest in between work.

2. DON'T IGNORE PAIN

During exercise or while working if you feel pain (more than usual) do not ignore it. Respect pain; change your activity if you feel pain. Thus stop activities if you feel that you are reaching a discomfort point. Limit activities which cause pain to last for half to one hour post activity. Excess pain may suggest active disease or joint damage. Do consult your doctor immediately.

3. BALANCED WORK

Too much rest increases the symptoms of RA. Too much work/activity increases the pain and can precipitate RA flare. Thus a balance needs to be created between work and rest so that RA symptoms remain in remission. Patient can rest before feeling tired. Adequate rest periods should be planned during difficult or long work.

4. ADEQUATE JOINT MOTION AND MUSCLE STRENGTH

Maintaining adequate joint range of motion and muscle strength is of prime importance for any patient of arthritis. Once range of motion and muscle strength start to decline the body functions decline too. Patients with RA should achieve full range of motion at each joint. Patients should also perform weight training to maintain muscle strength.

5. JUDICIOUS USE OF JOINTS

To perform tasks, patients with RA should work with unaffected joints as much as possible. Use of larger joints like shoulder, elbow, knee and hip makes work easy and comfortable for the patients. During the acute phase activities such as climbing stairs should be avoided.

6. AVOID PROLONGED POSITIONS

Keeping a joint in a particular position for a long time increases joint stiffness and hence joint pain. Thus, try to keep all the joints mobile and change positions. Getting up from your desk at regular intervals will help prevent joint and muscle stiffness.

7. WALK CAREFULLY

Rheumatoid arthritis patients have weak or osteoporotic bones. Fall poses big threat to sustain a fracture. So, these patients need to walk or do their activities very carefully. If the body moves well, stress on the joints can be prevented and hence the risk of fall decreases. Patients should not be in a hurry to do their work.

8.   MAINTAINING HEALTHY BODY WEIGHT

Healthy body weight prevents cardiovascular disease, keeps rheumatoid arthritis disease activity under control, and decreases the dose and amount of medicines used to treat RA. In addition, healthy weight decreases pressure and stress on joints and thus prolongs the life and efficacy of joints.

9.   WEAR SPLINTS/BRACE

Wearing a splint or a brace temporarily to offload the pressure on joints can prevent joint damage. Splints can be used to immobilize small joints so that rest can be given to the supportive structures.

HOW TO PROTECT HAND JOINTS

Hands and wrists are commonly affected joints in patients of RA. Hands are the most important structures by which we perform day to day activities. Hand and wrist protection need to be protected. Some ways to protect hand and wrist joints are –

a.   Use relaxed grip rather than a tight grasp. Release hand grip frequently if possible.
b.   Use of large diameter pens, utensils with thick handles can reduce pain of gripping. Use adaptive equipment such as jar openers.
c.   Use the palm of your hand to open the lid of a jar. Place the palm on the jar lid, and use body weight to turn your arm at shoulder.
d.   Avoid weight bearing on knuckles – it can damage the joints.
e.   Use both hands whenever possible.

f.   Avoid prolonged periods of hands in one position. Change position frequently to avoid joint stiffness. Release grip frequently while writing.

g.   Soak your hand in warm water to relieve pain.

h.   Use thick handled and long tooth brushes, spoons etc

i.   Large barrelled and rubber pens can be used for writing.

ACTIVITIES OF DAILY LIVING

•   Walking – people with walking issues may use walkers, stick etc

•   Climbing stairs – wearing foot, ankle, knee and back support may help some people

•   Kneeling, bending, stooping – avoid and use long handles instead

•   Good Grooming – use velcro and elastic rather than buttons, shoe laces etc

•   Hygiene – use high toilet seats, handlebars for support

•   Gripping – adaptive devices like built up door knobs and with levers etc

DO's

☐ DO rest for at least one hour in the afternoon when you begin to feel fatigued

☐ DO wear well fitted foot wear prescribed for you (absorb shock)

☐ DO use ice bag to reduce pain; apply a heating pad or take a hot shower to relax muscles before exercise

- DO use available devices to help you with dressing, bathing, cooking, working, and other activities
- DO make adjustments, at home and work, in your pace in completing tasks, to conserve energy
- DO apply for disability benefits if you are eligible or if you can no longer work
- DO perform muscle strengthening exercises once inflammation diminishes

DON'Ts

- DO NOT stay in bed longer than necessary
- DO NOT continue to wear an orthotic device that is uncomfortable or does not fit
- DO NOT overdo exercise. Daily exercise in small amounts is best
- DO NOT continue exercise if you feel pain after mild exercises – report to doctor
- DO NOT exercise a joint that is swollen
- DO NOT forget to exercise regularly when disease is in remission
- DO NOT stay at home all day; if you don't go out to work, be a volunteer or join an activities group
- DO NOT keep your fears and concerns about your health, or feelings of sadness or depression, to yourself. Talk to family, friends, or your doctor.

ROLE OF HOT AND COLD FOMENTATION IN RHEUMATOID ARTHRITIS PATIENTS

Hot and cold fomentation can decrease pain and stiffness in the joint, thus providing symptomatic relief to the patients. Warming the joints before exercising and applying cold after the exercise can ease the symptoms of joint pain and swelling.
Hot and cold fomentation has specific roles which are as follows-

Heat therapy for rheumatoid arthritis

Heat relaxes muscles, reduces the pain stiffness joints and increases blood flow and hence is useful for patients of rheumatoid arthritis. Heat therapy when combined with exercises increases the range of motion of joints.

Ways to use heat therapy –

1.   Warm bath or shower - soaking for 15 to 20 minutes in a warm bath allows the weight-bearing muscles to relax thus reducing pain and stiffness. To prolong the effect of a warm shower or bath, wear warm clothes.
2.   Moist heating pad
3.   Soaked damp folded towels dipped in hot water (to prevent burn, always test the temperature before using it).
4.   Paraffin bath – Can be used in consultation with a physiotherapist.

While applying heat therapy, use safe heat sources. To prevent burns, use heat for short lengths of time. One should be careful to check skin for redness while applying heat. If the redness occurs, the heat source should be removed. Always ask your doctor how to best use the heat therapy. .

Cold Therapy for Rheumatoid Arthritis

Cold therapy is generally used for inflamed joints. Cold therapy helps reduce inflammation, swelling, and soreness. It also relieves joint pain caused by an arthritis flare. Cold compresses reduce swelling by constricting blood vessels.

Ways to use cold therapy –

1.   Cold packs or gel packs or bag of frozen peas
2.   .Cooling the joints in cool water soak in a tub
3.   Cold sprays and ointments, such as biofreeze and cryoderm
4.   Ice wrapped in towel

If one suffers from Raynaud's syndrome (fingers or toes become red, blue or white when exposed to cold along with a feeling of pain or become numb) you should not use cold therapy. Ice or cold packs should not be directly applied to the skin, a towel or cloth between the cold device and the skin should always be used. To avoid frostbite, apply cold for less than 15 minutes at a time.

HOT AND COLD COMPRESSES WHEN AND WHAT TO DO

ACUTE CASES (joint pain & swelling)

        Cold therapy
Dosage
10 – 20 min/ 1-2 times a day

CHRONIC CASES (joint pain & swelling mild or nil)

Heat Therapy
Dosage
20 – 30 min - 1 to 2 times a day

CHAPTER 10

DIET MODIFICATIONS AND MAINTAINING ADEQUATE BODY WEIGHT IN PATIENTS WITH RHEUMATOID ARTHRITIS

Diet plays a major role in keeping a healthy body. Unbalanced diet is a risk factor of many diseases like diabetes, hypertension, deranged cholesterol, obesity, heart diseases, fatty liver and many more. Diet plays an important role in controlling the inflammatory response that is generated in patients of arthritis. Diet plays a major role in preventing disease flare and controlling disease. However, there are many myths prevailing in the society about which diet is beneficial and which is harmful. In this article I would put forth the scientific facts about the beneficial and harmful diet for patients with rheumatoid arthritis.
I would be discussing -

(I). DIETARY INTERVENTIONS USEFUL IN RHEUMATOID ARTHRITIS
(II). DIET THAT MAY INDUCE OR MAKE RHEUMATOID ARTHRITIS WORSE

(I). Dietary interventions useful in patients of RA –
Diets which have shown to be beneficial in arthritis
are as follow –

a)   VEGAN DIET
b)   SEVEN DAYS FASTING FOLLOWED BY
VEGAN DIET
c)   MEDITERRANEAN DIET
d)   ELIMINATION DIET
e)   DIETARY FIBRE AND WHOLE GRAINS
f)   FRUITS
g)   SPICES
h)   ESSENTIAL FATTY ACIDS
i)   GREEN TEA
j)   GLUTEN FREE DIET
k)   ANTI OXIDANTS
l)   Nuts

a)   VEGAN DIET
Intake of only fruits and vegetables, eliminating any
animal product or its by-products is a vegan diet.
Vegan diet has shown to decrease inflammation and
thus decrease arthritis activity. Studies claim that the
improvements in disease activity are the result of
reduction in immune-reactivity to certain food
antigens in the gastrointestinal tract that were
eliminated by adopting a vegan diet. Vegan diet also
plays an important role in many other diseases
especially patients with cancers.

b)   SEVEN DAYS FASTING FOLLOWED BY VEGAN DIET

It is proved that subtotal fasting with a limited amount of carbohydrate and energy along with vitamins and mineral supplementation and vegetable juice helps in reducing joint swelling, joint pain and inflammation. Fasting period of 7-10 days with partial nutrient intake in form of vegetable broth, herbal teas, garlic and decoction of potatoes, juice extracts from carrots, beets and celery. This has to be followed by controlled daily energy intake followed by 1 year of vegan diet decreases joint pain and swelling along with inflammatory markers as ESR and CRP.

c)   MEDITERRANEAN DIET
Mediterranean diet is rich in anti-inflammatory and antioxidant food. It consists of oleic acid, omega-3 fatty acids, unrefined carbohydrates, nuts, fruits, vegetables and plant products. Incorporating high amounts of olive oil, cereals, fruits, vegetables, fish, and legumes and moderate amounts of red wine in diet decreases joint pain, swelling and increases physical functions. Red meat, sweets and fried foods need to be avoided. Use of olive oil in diet decreases the risk of developing rheumatoid arthritis. Olive oil benefits joints as well as prevents heart diseases. Mediterranean diet has shown mixed results. Some studies have favored its role in RA; however some studies have not shown any decrease in inflammation. However, Mediterranean diet has all the anti-inflammatory and antioxidant properties and should benefit the patients of arthritis and autoimmune diseases.

d)   ELIMINATION DIET

Many patients complain that after eating certain food their arthritis symptoms worsened. Certain food and its components may worsen the disease. Thus, eliminate those food related antigens that may possibly aggravate the disease symptoms. Studies have shown that food allergens are one of the triggers of the immune system that increase inflammation and thus worsen symptoms of arthritis.

How to identify such antigens –

1.   Personal experience of foods that worsens arthritis

2.   Identifying allergen antigen by skin prick test

Eliminating allergen food for at least 8 weeks may be useful in controlling symptoms of arthritis.

e) DIETARY FIBRE AND WHOLE GRAIN CEREALS

Some studies found an inverse relationship between intake of dietary fiber and inflammatory biomarkers such as ESR & CRP which are indicators of inflammation in patients of rheumatoid arthritis. However, some studies did not find dietary fibers and whole grain cereals useful in reducing joint inflammation. Foods rich in whole grain and fiber are whole wheat, whole rice, oats, corn, rye, Barley, millets, Sorghum, canary seed, and wild rice. Whole grains provide rich amounts of antioxidants, phytic acid, vitamin E, selenium, many vitamins and minerals. These components are involved in anti-inflammatory processes and help the body in restoring inflammation to normal levels. Dietary fibers and whole grains are otherwise recommended for their health promotion. Thus, dietary fiber and whole grain cereals should be consumed regularly irrespective; a person is healthy or diseased.

f)   FRUITS AND VEGETABLES

Bioactive components and phytochemicals, present in fruits and vegetables have shown to decrease the symptoms of many diseases such as arthritis, diabetes, asthma and heart diseases. Regular consumption of fruits rich in phytochemicals reduces oxidative stress and inflammation. Fruits and plants with high anti oxidant and anti inflammatory properties are – avocados, dried plum, black rice, black soybean, grapefruits, banana, grapes, oranges, apples, cherries, blueberries and spinach. These fruits with anti inflammatory properties help in reducing inflammation in patients of RA. Vegetables are rich in phytochemicals, anti oxidants and contain anti inflammatory molecules.   Broccoli, spinach, advocado, cabbage, sprouts, bell peppers, carrots and mushrooms are some vegetables which have above mentioned properties.

g)   SPICES

Ginger, turmeric and cinnamon bark have proved to be useful as anti inflammatory agents both in rats and human studies. Turmeric has an active compound called curcumin which reduces joint pain and swelling. However, they need to be taken with warm substances as warm milk so as to increase the absorption of these substances and are absorbed in significant amounts to cause anti inflammatory action. Spices have also been used in traditional medicine for treating many diseases. Spices are generators of negative calories as they increase metabolic rate. Ginger and chillies are useful in this regard.

h)   ESSENTIAL FATTY ACIDS
Omega 3 fatty acid has a high anti-inflammatory property. They have shown to decrease joint pain and swelling in various types of arthritis including rheumatoid arthritis. Fish oils, flaxseed oil, walnut oil, mustard oil, olive oil, soybean oil, canola oil and corn oil are some of the oils rich in omega 3 fatty acid and have anti-inflammatory properties.

i)   GREEN TEA
Green tea has substances that have proven role in prevention and treatment of cardiovascular disease. It blocks inflammatory pathways and thus possesses anti-inflammatory properties. It is found to decrease joint swelling to some extent.

j)   GLUTEN FREE DIET

Gluten is a substance in certain foods like wheat which causes allergy and induces inflammation in the body. Scientific data regarding gluten free diet and its role in arthritis is inconclusive at the moment.

k)   ANTI OXIDANTS
Role of antioxidants like vitamin C, vitamin A, zinc and selenium in arthritis is doubtful. Some studies favour response while others do not.

I). NUTS
Nuts as almonds and walnuts have anti inflammatory properties and thus reduce inflammation in joints. Anti-inflammatory diet not only decreases body's inflammation but also increases energy levels in the body. Anti-inflammatory diet may help the patient to lose weight.

(II). Diet that may induce or make arthritis worse
Following list of food that are harmful in arthritis

a)   SWEETENED SUGAR SODA
b)   FRIED AND PROCESSED FOOD
c)   SUGAR AND REFINED CARBOHYDRATE
d)   SMOKING
e)   HIGH SALT AND PRESERVATIVES

a)   SUGAR SWEETENED SODA

Sweetened soda has been associated with an increased risk of rheumatoid arthritis. When compared to <1 sugar-sweetened soda per month, consumption of ≥1 sugar-sweetened soda per day has 63% increased risk of developing rheumatoid arthritis. Thus, sugar sweetened soda and products containing the same need to be avoided.

b)   FRIED AND PROCESSED FOOD
Decreasing fried and processed foods shall reduce inflammation and help restore the body's natural defence.

c)   SUGARS AND REFINED CARBOHYDRATE
High amounts of sugar in diet can cause inflammation in the body and worsen arthritis symptoms. Thus, the same needs to be avoided in the diet.

d)   SMOKING
Smoking not only increases the risk of heart attacks and cancers, it also increases the risk of development of rheumatoid arthritis. People with arthritis who smoke are at risk of lung involvement. Smoking is highly prohibited in patients with arthritis.

e)   HIGH SALT AND PRESERVATIVE RICH DIET
Some studies suggest that diet rich in salt and preservatives worsen inflammation and thus worsen arthritis.

ANTI-INFLAMMATORY DIET SHOULD CONTAIN –

1. 25 gram of fiber per day
2. 2 servings of fruits and 7 servings of vegetables (1 serving = equates to half a cup of fruit or cooked vegetables or one cup of raw leafy vegetables)
3. Whole grain cereals
4. Avoid alcohol
5. EAT FOUR SERVINGS OF ALLIUMS AND CRUCIFERS WEEKLY (Alliums include garlic, scallions, onions and leeks, while crucifers refer to vegetables such as broccoli, cabbage, cauliflower, mustard greens and Brussels sprouts)
6. Consume omega 3 rich foods
7. Cook with herbs and spices
8. Avoid processed food and sugars
9. Avoid saturated fats and trans fats
10. .Use unsaturated fats and oils

CONCLUSION

In nutshell, one should stick to the anti inflammatory diet - must include more fruits and vegetables, avoid fried and sugary foods. Alcohol needs to be avoided, smoking is totally prohibited. One should maintain healthy weight and do regular exercise. There is no fixed diet plan that is proven for RA patients. What works for one person may not work for others. Hit, trial and error help one determine which foods one need to remove from diet. The role of diet has its limitations. It cannot replace the role of medications. It has proven benefits but as an adjunct to medications. Definitely, it may decrease the amount and dose of medicines by decreasing inflammation and thus decreasing disease activity. However, before starting a new diet or food a patient should consult his/her doctor as dietary changes can lead to negative interaction with medicines.

MAINTAINING ADEQUATE BODY WEIGHT
Weight management is an important part of everyone's life. People who maintain the right weight for their age and height mostly enjoy a healthy life. They are less prone for serious diseases like diabetes, heart attacks etc. Similarly, weight management plays a very important role in management of RA patients.

IMPORTANCE OF WEIGHT LOSS IN RA
•   Reduce pressure on your joints thus reduce pain
•   Reduce inflammation in body and joints
•   Reduce Disease Activity in RA
•   Reduces risk of RA flare

- Slows Cartilage Degeneration in joints
- Decreases dose/number of medicines
- Reduces risk of comorbidities such as diabetes, heart disease.

WAYS TO ACHIEVE ADEQUATE WEIGHT IN RA

1. Avoid fast food, fried products, bakery products, sweets or sugary products.
2. Diet should be rich in proteins, fruits, green leafy vegetables, salad and fibers (unless contraindicated).
3. Coffee intake helps in weight loss as caffeine stimulates the nervous system to break fat cells in our body.
4. Drink water between meals as it increases the body's metabolism and helps lose weight.
5. Take 3 meals a day. Avoid eating post sunset and no late night meals. Last meal of the day should be very less in amount.
6. Eat whole food rather than processed food. The amount of food that you put on your plate should be reduced by 25 percent or take 3-4 tablespoon off your plate.
7. Exercise for 30-45 minutes a day. However, one should do only those exercises which are feasible. Cycling, walking, swimming and aerobics are good exercises which not only help in weight loss but also prevent cardiovascular diseases.

CHAPTER 11

QUALITY OF LIFE IN RHEUMATOID ARTHRITIS & WAYS TO IMPROVE IT

Quality of life as defined by the World Health Organization (WHO) means, "individual's perception of their position in life in terms of culture and systems in which they live, in relation to their goals, expectations, standards and concerns".

Quality of life includes - physical health, psychological state, level of independence, social relationships, personal beliefs and their relationships. Rheumatoid arthritis affects multidimensional aspects of life. RA affects the physical health due to joint pain and deformities. Patients often are not able to perform everyday tasks. RA also affects emotional and psychological aspects of life. Changes in self-perception in relation to painful stimuli, reduced functional ability, and labour and social inadequacy may also induce emotional and mental disorders.

As RA affects multiple domains of life thus quality of life questionnaires in RA include all those domains. Quality of life questionnaires in RA include - the physical dimensions (pain and deterioration of physical functioning), the psychological dimension (anxiety and depression), the cognitive dimension (attention and memory) and the social dimension (self-esteem and interpersonal relationships).

STRATEGIES TO IMPROVE QUALITY OF LIFE IN RA PATIENTS

1.	Disease acceptance – It has been seen in studies that the patients who accept the disease and start living with it have better quality of life then those who don't accept the disease as a part of themselves. Thus, accepting disease early and starting treatment prevents joint damage and hence prevents deterioration of quality of life.

2.	Early treatment – Early diagnosis and treatment prevents joint deformities, less risk of developing depression and anxiety. Patients are able to do all the activities related to personal and professional life.

3.	Achieving low disease activity – Low disease activity or disease under control is associated with better quality of life then patients with moderate to severe disease activity.

4.	Empowering patients of RA - Empowerment helps the patients think critically to have the opportunity to make autonomous and informed decisions so they can get what they need, handle everyday life and enhance quality of life. The empowered patients used their knowledge of having had a long-term condition for several years, and had a belief in their own ability to manage different situations, and how to reset goals and expectations. Empowering a patient of RA helps improve the quality of life of the patients.

5.	Social support - Accessibility of different social relationships and participation with family, friends and colleagues improves quality of life of patients with RA

6.   Continuing professional - Continuing the professional work and keeping ones engaged improves the quality of life of patients.

7.   Sleep – Disturbed or inadequate sleep is associated with poor quality of life as compared to patients with a normal sleep pattern.

8.   Anxiety & depression – Patients with RA who develop anxiety and depression lead poor quality of life. However, once both these problems are under control the quality of life of a RA patient improves.

9.   Emergency health funds – RA patients may develop health emergencies at some point in their life. Thus, some amount of money should be kept aside as an emergency fund.

DISEASE ACCEPTANCE

Acceptance is considered as adjustment, adaptation or negotiation with chronic pain. It becomes very important to accept the disease because acceptance is the first step to control disease/chronic pain.
Sequences in accepting a chronic disease include - becoming aware of the problem and receiving a diagnosis; acknowledging the chronicity of the pain and the resulting losses; and establishing a new way of living.

Studies have shown that disease acceptance plays a positive role in patients' physical, social and emotional functioning. It has been seen in various studies that the patients who come to terms with pain report more positive clinical outcomes, greater confidence in their coping ability, higher daily uptime, less depression and less pain. They respond better to treatment and live a better quality of life.

Earlier the acceptance, the better it is for the patients with RA. Accepting the disease early and starting regular treatment prevents joint damage and hence prevents surgery or complications of rheumatoid arthritis.

It has been seen that the higher the level of disease acceptance, the more self sufficient and active the patient is. The patients who have accepted their condition generally accept the necessity of treatment and also trust their medical personnel. By not accepting the disease, one risks making things much worse for oneself.

Thus, disease acceptance plays an important role in chronic diseases like rheumatoid arthritis. Patients who accept the disease early do well as compared to patients who accept the disease late.

Tips to Help one Accept the Life Changes in RA

Arthritis makes a lot of changes in the body. One should adapt to the changes else it will make things worse for the patient. Tips to adapt to RA are -

1. Recognize your physical limitations and remember your true ability
2. Do not feel guilty if you need help
3. Must cancel plans if you are not well
4. Be kind and gentle to yourself
5. Remember the consequences of any wrongdoing
6. Accept your new reality
7. Safety first should be the approach

CHAPTER 12

REAL LIFE SCENARIOS OF RHEUMATOID ARTHRITIS PATIENTS

There are many real life case summaries of patients which tell us the importance of early diagnosis and regular treatment in rheumatoid arthritis. I would be sharing such stories so that people are motivated and do not lose hope.

Case1
- Patient A – age – 42 yrs, beginning of RA symptoms since 1 year
- On regular treatment and follow up for 7 years
- Currently – no joint damage or any organ involvement, living a healthy normal life, only on 2 medicines per day, going to office

Lesson learnt – Early diagnosis and regular treatment help preserve joints, risk of involvement of major organs of the body like heart, brain, lung, etc decreases, patients require less medicines to control disease and patient is able to perform all his household and professional work independently.

Case 2
- Patient B –32 years age, beginning of RA symptoms since 1 year
- Was doing well on medicines, left treatment as she wanted medicine free disease control
- Visited after 7 years – mild to moderate deformities and joint damage

- Had lung involvement
- Requires multiple medicines including biologicals and oxygen therapy for lung involvement

Lesson learnt – Patient was diagnosed early and was doing well on medicines. Patient left treatment developed joint damage and lung involvement. Patient required biological therapy along with multiple medicines and oxygen later on.

Case 3

- Patient C- 40 years age, Disease duration – 10 years – irregular treatment
- Severe joint damage – would require knee joint replacement
- Developed stroke or paralysis due RA

Lesson learnt – irregular treatment leads to joint damage and increases the risk of paralysis due to swelling/inflammation in blood vessels due to RA

Case 4

- Case of RA age 50 years – 15 years disease duration – did not take proper treatment - knee replaced – doing well on medicines – post surgery – doing all her activities, going to office
- Living a healthy life with medicines

Lesson learnt – Irregular treatment leads to uncontrolled disease which can damage joints. Once joints are severely damaged surgery will be required. Patients can lead a healthy independent life post knee replacement with medicines for RA alone.

Case 5

- Case of RA – age – 28 years, disease symptoms since 5 years, patient on regular treatment since 5 years taking oral medicines. However, diseases still not controlled with oral medicines, patients require biological therapy. Patient agrees for the same, given biological therapy.
- Patient's disease is fully under control. Better response to oral medicines and biological therapy stopped.

Lesson learnt – Biological therapy when used at right time can control the disease and hence prevent joint damage.

Case 6

- 35 yr male – RA since 5 years
- Initially wrist and hands involved – became better with medicines – left treatment – pain swelling restarted – took pain killers – after 6 months visited clinic again as disease became severe and spread to all joints – started medicines – became better after 6 months – self medicating – came after 1 year with lung involvement and joints requiring replacements and biological therapy. Patient also developed diabetes.

Lesson learnt – Irregular treatment leads to uncontrolled disease which can damage joints and lungs. Such patients may require higher therapy as biological. RA if uncontrolled poses a huge risk of developing diabetes, heart attacks etc.

Case 7

- RA since 10 years – irregular and delayed treatment – knee joints damaged – replaced (3.5 lacs), lung involved – required frequent hospitalization due to lung infections or breathing difficulties, require costly medicines for treatment

Lesson learnt – Irregular and delayed treatment causes uncontrolled disease which possesses risk of joint damage and recurrent hospitalisations due to increased risk of infections due to uncontrolled RA.

Case 8
- 43 year female, case of RA – total disease duration since 7 years on methotrexate, hydroxychloroquine, sulfasalazine, leflunomide and low dose steroids
- Disease moderately active despite above medicines
- Patient obese with weight of 85 kg and BMI of 30.2 kg/m sq
- Patient lost weight – current weight of 67 kg, BMI of 23.7 kg/msq
- RA in spontaneous remission, now disease control with only methotrexate once a week

Lesson learnt – weight loss plays a major role in management of RA

Case 9
36 year female with RA since 4 years – with no other disease – not taking proper treatment for RA – after 2 years develops diabetes and increased blood pressure.

Lesson Learnt – Untreated or uncontrolled RA patients are at increased risk of developing other diseases as diabetes, increased blood pressure, blood cancers etc.

Case 10

42 year old male, smoker, case of RA on treatment with disease under good control with medicines suddenly develops prolonged dry cough – on evaluation found to have interstitial lung disease.

Lesson learnt – RA patients who are smokers have increased risk of lung involvement in RA.

CHAPTER 13

IMPORTANCE OF REGULAR VISITS TO A DOCTOR

Many times a patient thinks why to visit a doctor when he/she is doing fine. But, it is very important to visit a doctor regularly as he advises due to multiple reasons –

1.Doctors need to check whether the disease is completely under control or is progressive.

2.Every doctor has a plan for each of his/her patients to minimize the amount of medicine when a patient is doing well on a particular set of medicine.

3.During each visit a doctor needs to check whether his/her patient is developing side effects or complications (involvement of heart, lung, kidney, nerves, eyes etc) of disease. If that complication is detected early it shall be reversed completely.

4.During each visit a doctor checks whether his/her patient develops any side effects of medicines or not.

5.The doctor checks whether the patient is developing any comorbidity like diabetes, high blood pressure, obesity, heart problems etc.

6.Time to time, a doctor advises the lifestyle modifications for his/her patients.

Thus by visiting your doctor regularly, you can avoid hospitalizations as complications can be detected early and can be reversed on OPD basis only. Visiting your doctor regularly you can minimize the medicines and prevent joint damage. It has been seen that patients who don't visit their doctor regularly are the ones who develop more side effects of medicines then those who regularly visits their doctor. Thus, a patient must visit his/her doctor on a regular basis to avoid above complications.

CHAPTER 14

MEDICINES TO TREAT RHEUMATOID ARTHRITIS PATIENTS

With advancement in medical science, there is tremendous advancement in the management of rheumatoid arthritis. Gold and penicillamine which were once considered gold standard for the treatment for RA have become things of the past. Newer and safer medicines are available to treat patients of RA. Newer medicines are more efficacious and have less side effects though cost of those medicines is still a concern in most of the places.

An important thing is – one medicine may work well for one patient and may not work for another the same way. Sometimes it may take a year or two for the doctor to find which medicine best suits a particular patient. Give your doctor time to find out what works best for you.

Medicines used to treat RA are -

- Anti inflammatory medicines – Non steroidal anti inflammatory drugs - NSAIDS (pain killers), Steroids
- Traditional DMARDs (Disease modifying anti rheumatic drugs)- Methotrexate, Leflunomide, hydroxychloroquine, Sulfasalazine
- Biological DMARDs - TNF blockers (infliximab, eternacept, golimumab, adalimumab), Tocilizumab, Rituximab, Abatacept

- Oral biological - Tofacitinib, Baricitinib
- Iguratimod
- Immunosuppressant drugs - Mycophenolate mofetil, Azathioprine, Cyclophosphamide, Tacrolimus

1.   Anti inflammatory medicines -

This class of medicines comprise of medicines which are helpful for the patients in active or flare up of RA. This class of drugs are used till the time the main DMARDs start acting. The medicines in this class are slowly tapered off and can be used again when disease flares up. These medicines are to be used wisely by the treating doctor.

2.   Traditional DMARDs (Disease modifying anti rheumatic drugs)-

This class of medicines used to treat RA includes – methotrexate, sulfasalazine, leflunomide and hydroxychloroquine. These medicines as the name suggests are disease modifying that is they stop disease progression of RA. They not only stop disease progression but also prevent RA patients from infections by controlling the disease. They also prevent RA patients from getting extra articular manifestations like heart attack, stroke etc. These medicines are slow to act and take 3-6 months to reach full effect.

3.   Biological DMARDs

Biological DMARDs is a class of drugs which are modern medicines with high efficacy to control RA. These drugs generally act quickly and control disease in a way that they stop disease progression. These medicines are generally indicated when traditional DMARDs fail to control the disease activity. These medicines are a bit costly injectable medicines which can be given by intravenous route or subcutaneous route. The medicines in this group comprise of –

a)   TNF Blockers – Adalimumab and its biosimilars, Infliximab and its biosimilars, Golimumab, eternacept and its biosimilars
b)   IL-6 inhibitor – Tocilizumab
c)   IL-1 inhibitor – Anakinra
d)   Fusion molecule – Abatacept
e)   B cell depletion - Rituximab

4.   JAK KINASE INHIBITORS

These are relatively newer classes of oral tablets which have dramatically changed the management of RA. These medicines are highly efficacious medicines to treat RA.

5.   IGURATIMOD

This is a new class of medicine used to treat patients of rheumatoid arthritis. This medicine is however not approved to be used in all countries.

6.   IMMUNOSUPPRESSANT DRUGS

Immunosuppressant medicines in RA play a major role when RA has spread beyond joints. These are helpful when RA has involved lungs, eyes, kidneys, brain and nerves etc. Medicines in this class include mycophenolate mofetil, cyclosporine, cyclophosphamide, tacrolimus and azathioprine.

WHEN AND HOW MUCH RESPONSE TO EXPECT IN RA

Response to treatment in rheumatoid arthritis depends on multiple factors – most important of which is how early the treatment has been initiated after starting of disease symptoms.

Other factors depend upon the degree of joint damage, the physical functional status of the patient, psychological health, and the presence of comorbid illness such as cardiovascular disease, infection, and B cell lymphomas.

Treatment response in general is slow in patients of RA. It is expected that the majority of patients would take 3-6 months to get the symptoms to normalise. It is to be considered that 30-40 percent of patients won't respond to the normal (conventional/traditional DMARDs) medicines used to treat RA. In these patients higher therapy as biological DMARDs or JAK kinase inhibitors need to be added.

Moreover, an important thing for the patient to note is not all patients respond to the same medicines. Also, not all patients respond equally to all medicines. Doctors need to find out which is the best cocktail of medicine that will be the most effective for a patient. Sometimes to find out the same, it may take months to a year or two.

It has been shown that a 33% reduction of radiographic/disease progression in patients of RA who was treated earlier than 2 years disease duration compared with those treated later. These benefits were sustained up to 5 years.

Long term outcome (10 year) of treated patients with early arthritis (less than 2 year duration) was assessed in multiple studies. 94 percent of those treated early and regularly were able to do all their functions by themselves at 10 years.

Response is sustained in those patients who are on regular treatment rather than taking intermittent medicines.

SIDE EFFECTS OF MEDICINES TO TREAT RHEUMATOID ARTHRITIS

Rheumatoid arthritis is a controllable disease. Medicines are an essential element to control disease activity of RA. If the disease remains uncontrolled it shall damage the joints and cause disability and deformity. Not only joints, uncontrolled disease may damage important organs of the body like heart, brain, lungs, nerves, eyes etc. These side effects of disease will occur in almost 100 percent of the patients of RA if the disease remains untreated.

Medicines used to treat RA are essential to control disease activity. As said – nothing is 100 percent safe in this universe. Neither the food we eat (food can cause infection and many other diseases), nor the medicines. There is a risk of airplanes getting crashed when we travel. Similarly, the medicines are not 100 percent safe. However, these medicines to treat RA have been studied in animals and humans and the side effect of these medicines is well known. These side effects don't occur in every individual. Serious side effects of these medicines are rare and occur in 1 in thousands or lacs of patients. There are ways to monitor these side effects of medicines used to treat RA. By regular monitoring, we can detect these side effects early and can be easily reversed.

I will be discussing some side effects of medicines used to treat RA along with measures by which we can avoid side effects of medicines.

MEDICINES	SIDE EFFECTS	WATCH OUT FOR	MONITORING/PRECAUTIONS

| NSAIDs | Gastrointestinal ulceration and bleeding, renal damage etc | Blood in stool, dyspepsia, nausea or vomiting, weakness, dizziness, abdominal pain, edema, weight, gain, shortness of breath | Liver function tests (LFT), kidney function tests(KFT) and urinalysis within 3 months - repeat these studies every 6 to 12 months if low risk or every 3 monthly if high risk (to be decided by doctor) |

Corticosteroid	Hypertension, Hyperglycemia, cataract, weight gain, Osteoporosis, infections, gastric ulcers etc	Symptoms of frequent urination, increased thirst, edema, visual changes, weight gain, nausea, vomiting, headaches, broken bones or bone pain	Vaccinations as per your doctor, 3 monthly check up for sugar, weight control, regular exercise, yearly eye check up, blood pressure monitoring
Methotrexate	Nausea, vomiting, Bone marrow suppression, Increased liver enzymes, hepatic fibrosis, cirrhosis, alopecia,	Shortness of breath, nausea or vomiting, lymph node swelling, coughing, oral ulcers, diarrhea, hair fall, jaundice	Vaccinations as per your doctor, blood tests as Complete blood count (CBC), LFT, KFT initially monthly for 3 months then every 3 monthly

	stomatitis, rash, infections etc		
Leflunomide	Increased liver enzymes , gastrointestinal distress, bone marrow suppression, alopecia, infections etc	Nausea or vomiting, gastritis, diarrhea, hair loss, weight loss, oral ulcers, loose stools, jaundice	Vaccinations as per your doctor, blood tests as CBC, LFT, KFT initially monthly for 3 months then every 3 monthly

Sulfasalazine	Bone marrow suppression, Rash, abdominal pain, headache etc	Abdomen pain, headache, photosensitivity, rash, nausea or vomiting	Blood tests as CBC, LFT, KFT initially monthly for 3 months then every 3 monthly
Hydroxychloroquine	Dark skin, rash, itching, diarrhea, rarely deposition in eye etc	Visual changes including a decrease in night or peripheral vision, rash, diarrhea	Yearly eye check up by an ophthalmologist

Etanercept, Adalimumab, Anakinra Infliximab, Rituximab, Abatacept	Local injection-site reactions, infections, Immune reactions etc	Symptoms of infection like fever, prolonged cough, parasthesia, postinfusion reactions etc	Vaccinations and blood tests as per your doctor
Tofacitinib, baricitinib	Herpes zoster, Herpes simplex, Gastroenteritis, Urinary tract infections, thrombocytosis, nausea etc	Fever, skin rash, abdomen pain, vomiting etc	Vaccinations and blood tests as per your doctor

Mycophenolate mofetil	Abdomen pain, decreased leucocyte count, infections	Watch out for increased frequency of stools, abdomen pain, loose stool, vomiting, hair fall, etc	Vaccinations as per your doctor

In general, mild side effects are relatively common but are easily reversible. Major side effects are very rare and can be averted by regular monitoring and precautions which your doctor advises. Remember, the side effects of RA are much more dangerous and irreversible than the medicines used to treat it.

The most important step to avoid side effects of disease or medicines is to follow your doctor regularly. It has been seen that side effects of disease or medicines occur in those patients who do not visit their doctor regularly or don't follow instructions of their doctor. Doctor examines his/her patients and orders tests from time to time to keep a check on side effects of medicines used to treat RA.

To realize the importance of medicines to treat RA let us know what may happen if we don't take any medicine.

The disease RA if left untreated shall experience progressive symptoms (may progress slowly or quickly) and damage the bones, cartilage, and other structures of the joints. Joint damage will typically worsens over time and is irreversible and impact's person's routine activities, and leads to significant disability. Not only that, untreated RA can involve major organs of the body like heart, brain, kidney & lungs. Life expectancy is near normal in regularly treated patients however in untreated or irregular treated it is 15 years short.

Thus, untreated RA will have more side effects than the medicines itself.

CHAPTER 15

BLUEPRINT TO A PAIN FREE LIFE AMONGST PATIENTS WITH RHEUMATOID ARTHRITIS

Rheumatoid arthritis is a chronic disease requiring lifelong treatment in most of the cases. As discussed in previous chapters it is combined effort from both doctor & patient that can change the life of RA patient to a pain free life. I shall be discussing the steps a RA patient should follow to live a pain free life.

STEPS WHICH A PATIENT SUFFERING FROM RHEUMATOID ARTHRITIS MUST FOLLOW TO LIVE A PAIN FREE LIFE -

1.   First and foremost thing which a patient of RA must recognize is that he/she suffers from a disease called rheumatoid arthritis. This disease is incurable just like most other diseases (diabetes, increased blood pressure, thyroid disorders, kidney, heart, lung diseases etc). However, incurable does not mean that there is no treatment available for the same. There are good and advanced medicines which are now easily available that can control the disease and prevent complications. Thus, disease acceptance is the foremost & most important step.

2.   Second step towards a pain free life is to visit a specialist for RA treatment. Rheumatologists are specialists who are properly trained to treat RA.

3.   It has been seen that the patients who start treatment early are able to live painless or life with mild pain as compared to patients who delay their treatment or have developed deformities or complications. So, starting early is the key to living a pain free life.

4.   Further, trusting your doctor is the next step. Your doctor shall prescribe you medicines depending on the stage of your disease. Sometimes biological therapy may be required to control the disease. He/she may order tests on a regular interval to look for side effects of disease or medicines.

5.   Following proper lifestyle modifications play an important role in controlling the disease. Once a patient adjusts his/her life accordingly, then only he/she may be able to achieve pain free life.
Lifestyle modifications which a patient of RA must follow are – regular exercise, maintaining adequate body weight, eating a balanced anti inflammatory diet, taking adequate timely sleep, following joint protection techniques and activities of daily living.
6.   Patients suffering from rheumatoid arthritis are at increased risk of developing psychiatric manifestations as depression and anxiety. These aspects need to be managed properly with self motivation techniques as described in this book. If self motivation techniques aren't adequate to control psychiatric manifestations then patients need to consult a doctor for the same.

7.   Controlling co morbid illness as thyroid diseases, diabetes, heart diseases etc help reduce pain in the body. Adequately controlling co morbid illness plays an important role in living a pain free life.

8.   Regular follow up is another major aspect of treatment of RA. It has been seen that those patients who follow their doctor regularly are at less risk of developing side effects of disease or the medicines. The disease in these patients gets controlled early and requires fewer medicines.

In short it has to be a regular sustained effort from both doctor and patient which enables one to live a pain free life amongst patients with rheumatoid arthritis.

SUMMARY

To summarize, rheumatoid arthritis is a disease which can easily spread beyond joints. RA can occur at any age but the most common age is 3rd to 4th decade. Untreated RA can damage joints and lead to deformities. Untreated RA can spread to major organs like heart, lungs, kidneys, nerves, blood vessels etc. Patients with untreated or uncontrolled disease are at risk of premature death in RA.

Lifestyle modifications like exercise, weight reduction, joint protection, diet etc plays a major role and are adjunct to medicines in treating RA. Patients with RA are at increased risk of psychological complications like anxiety, depression and insomnia. Self management of psychological complications along with medicines (if required) not only controls psychological health but also pain and improves quality of life of RA patients.

Early and regular treatment of RA not only prevents joint damage but also prevents economic burden to the patient as the patient is able to continue his/her work to earn livelihood.

Medicines are the mainstay in treating RA patients. Earlier you start the treatment the better it is in terms of disease control as well as medicine requirements. However in some cases, patients do not respond to simple conventional DMARDs and require higher therapy as biological which controls the disease very quickly and efficiently. The joints which are destroyed require replacement or surgical intervention by an orthopedician.

Most important aspect in RA management is regular follow up with a rheumatologist. Patients who follow their doctor regularly generally have well controlled disease, require fewer medicines with time, live better quality of life and generally don't develop side effects of disease or medicines.

In short, RA treatment requires a dual effort by patient and doctor so that the patient lives a good quality pain free life.

Manufactured by Amazon.ca
Acheson, AB

17182686R00063